Felipe Q. S. Guerra
Mariana Morais Sá
Julio A. Pereira

Invasive Aspergillosis - Diagnosis and Recommended Therapy

Felipe Q. S. Guerra
Mariana Morais Sá
Julio A. Pereira

Invasive Aspergillosis - Diagnosis and Recommended Therapy

Literature review on invasive aspergillosis and diagnostic and therapeutic difficulties

ScienciaScripts

Cover image: www.ingimage.com

This book is a translation from the original published under ISBN 978-613-9-70417-0.

Publisher:
Sciencia Scripts
is a trademark of
Dodo Books Indian Ocean Ltd. and OmniScriptum S.R.L publishing group

120 High Road, East Finchley, London, N2 9ED, United Kingdom
Str. Armeneasca 28/1, office 1, Chisinau MD-2012, Republic of Moldova, Europe
Printed at: see last page
ISBN: 978-620-8-20380-1

SUMMARY

Aspergillosis, an infection caused by fungal species of the genus *Aspergillus*, has emerged as a highly important disease in intensive care units in hospitals, with invasive aspergillosis being the disease with the highest levels of mortality and morbidity. The genus *Aspergillus* is distributed worldwide and in various habitats, with no geographical predilection. The *A. fumigatus* species is the aetiological agent responsible for approximately 90% of cases of aspergillosis. Aspergillosis encompasses a wide spectrum of diseases, in which it can manifest itself in various ways, whether through allergic diseases, chronic cavitary forms or invasive disease. Invasive aspergillosis is considered an opportunistic, progressive, acute and severe fungal infection, with a poor prognosis and the greatest risk to life in immunosuppressed patients or those who are subject to extremely aggressive therapies using corticoids, antibiotics and immunosuppressive drugs, as well as in cases of prolonged agranulocytosis. Invasive aspergillosis is difficult to diagnose, its symptoms and clinical signs are non-specific and appear late in the infection, making early diagnosis very important. It is of great importance that treatment is started as soon as possible, thus generating a better prognosis. Voriconazole is the drug recommended as first-line therapy, as it has been shown to have better efficacy and tolerance compared to amphotericin B.

Keywords: *Aspergillus* spp. Invasive aspergillosis. Clinical aspects. Diagnosis. Therapeutics.

CONTENTS

CHAPTER 1

INTRODUCTION

Mycology comprises a vast field of study involving micro-organisms known as fungi and yeasts (OLIVEIRA, 2014). Over time, more than 100,000 species of fungi have been recognised and described. However, fewer than 500 of these species have been linked to diseases in humans, and no more than 100 species are capable of causing infection in healthy individuals. The rest are only capable of causing disease in debilitated or immunocompromised individuals (KAUFFMAN et al., 2011).

However, due to the prolonged survival of patients with multiple risk factors for fungal infections, such as haematopoietic stem cell transplantation, solid organ transplantation, new chemotherapy agents and immunosuppressants, the number of systemic fungal infections has increased by approximately 207% in recent decades (LAI et al., 2008; ALANGADEN, 2011; APERIS; ALIVANIS, 2011; ROBBINS et al., 2011). Among these, hospital-acquired infections are the most important, as their progressive increase has contributed to a greater rise in morbidity and mortality rates (MARTINS-DINIZ et al., 2005).

Aspergillosis, an infection caused by fungal species of the genus *Aspergillus*, has emerged as a highly important disease in intensive care units in hospitals, with invasive aspergillosis being the disease with the highest levels of mortality and morbidity (MEERSSEMAN et al., 2007).

The genus *Aspergillus* has around 339 accepted species (SAMSON et al., 2014) and is widely distributed in nature, particularly in the air, decaying organic material, soil, water, food, surfaces and ventilation systems. In addition to their wide distribution, fungi of the genus *Aspergillus* have enteroblastic conidiogenesis of the phialidic type, with a high capacity for sporulation. In atmospheric air we find around 1-100 conidia per m^3 (BULPA et al., 2007).

Inhaling *Aspergillus* spores *is* the usual way for humans to develop the infection, and the incubation period is still unknown. In the lungs, the spores originate hyphae that can invade nearby tissues or even other organs; however, the consequences of inhaling these spores depend essentially on the individual's immune status (PARTRIDGE- HINCKLEY et al., 2009; ASKEW; KONTOYIANNIS; CLEMONS, 2014).

In immunocompetent people, after inhalation of the conidia by the host, the spores are normally eliminated by the activity of alveolar macrophages, where this process often occurs without impairing body homeostasis or the manifestation of specific symptoms (GUAZZELLI et al., 2012; BARBERÁN; MENSA, 2014).

In immunocompromised patients, inhalation of fungal spores can cause lung diseases ranging from local airway inflammation to severe, life-threatening lung infections such as allergic bronchopulmonary aspergillosis and invasive aspergillosis (BEISSWENGER et al., 2012).

Aspergillosis encompasses a wide spectrum of diseases, in which it can manifest itself in various ways, both through allergic diseases (allergic fungal rhinosinusitis, allergic bronchopulmonary aspergillosis, severe asthma with hypersensitivity to fungi and extrinsic allergic alveolitis), as well as chronic cavitary forms (which usually involve immunocompetent patients who have previous structural damage to the lung parenchyma) or can also manifest as invasive disease (which can progress rapidly or have a subacute or even chronic course, depending on the patient's immunity). (DENNING, 2010, WINGARD; HSU, 2010). In recent years, there has been great concern about invasive aspergillosis, as its occurrence has increased, particularly in individuals with severely compromised immune systems (PAULUSSEN et al., 2016).

Invasive aspergillosis is considered an opportunistic, progressive, acute and severe fungal infection, with a poor prognosis and the greatest risk to life in immunosuppressed patients or those who are subject to extremely aggressive therapies through the use of corticoids, antibiotics and immunosuppressive drugs, as well as in cases of prolonged agranulocytosis, and its most common form is pulmonary invasive aspergillosis, which is characterised by the proliferation of aspergillus forms in the lung parenchyma (RAJA; SINGH, 2006; DAGENAIS; KELLER, 2009; KOUSHA; TADI; SOUBANI 2011; KOSMIDIS; DENNING, 2015). It is also possible for the fungus to spread from the lungs to the gastrointestinal tract, kidneys, brain, liver or other organs, causing abscesses and necrotic lesions (PERSON et al., 2010).

Invasive aspergillosis is difficult to diagnose, its symptoms and clinical signs are nonspecific and appear late in the infection, making early diagnosis very important. The appearance of persistent fever, the only sign of infection, and the existence of non-specific or attenuated symptoms as a result of corticosteroid medication, make diagnosis difficult, due to the lack of a diagnostic method capable of identifying the fungus responsible for the infection, treatment is not carried out in the appropriate time, which may be associated with high mortality rates, with the diagnosis being confirmed by autopsy (DIMOPOULOS et al., 2010).

When not treated appropriately, invasive pulmonary aspergillosis can easily worsen, leading to dissemination to the central nervous system, heart, veins or other structures close to the lung (ALDERSON et al., 2005; CADENA et al., 2016).

In invasive pulmonary aspergillosis, it is of great importance that treatment is started as soon as possible, thus generating a better prognosis (CADENA et al., 2016). Voriconazole is the drug recommended as first-line therapy, as it has been shown to have better efficacy and tolerance compared to amphotericin B (BADDLEY et al., 2013; JACOBS et al., 2011).

In view of the above, there is great concern on the part of health professionals about invasive infections, since the mortality rate is high and there is still a delay in truly effective forms of diagnosis. There are currently few review studies available on the subject, but in view of the above, it is clear how important it is to know about invasive aspergillosis and the factors surrounding this disease, such as the mode of contamination, risk factors, diagnosis and treatment; therefore, it is necessary to frequently carry out current review studies on the subject.

CHAPTER 2

OBJECTIVES

2.1 GENERAL

- To carry out a literature review on the clinical, laboratory and therapeutic factors of invasive aspergillosis.

2.2 SPECIFIC

- Describe the etiological and epidemiological aspects of the *Aspergillus* genus;
- Discuss the clinical characteristics of invasive aspergillosis;
- Outline up-to-date diagnostic and therapeutic methods for invasive aspergillosis;

CHAPTER 3

METHODOLOGY

This research is characterised as a narrative review, where the criteria used to search and critically analyse the literature are not explicit and systematic. A narrative review allows knowledge on a given topic to be obtained and updated in a short space of time; however, it does not have a methodology that enables data to be reproduced, nor does it provide quantitative answers to certain questions (ROTHER, 2007).

The inclusion criteria used to select the studies in this narrative review were: theses, books and scientific articles on the subject available in databases and search engines, productions in Portuguese and English, and publications between 2007 and 2017.

The exclusion criteria for the articles were book chapters, dissertations, theses and scientific articles that did not have the full text available online and that did not cover the proposed topic and designated period.

The guiding question of this study was: "What are the various factors related to invasive aspergillosis?". The bibliographic survey was carried out between January and April 2018.

The terms used to search for the articles were: aspergillosis, clinical aspects, diagnosis, epidemiology, treatment. And their respective English translations: Aspergillosis, clinical aspects, diagnosis, epidemiology, treatment.

CHAPTER 4

NARRATIVE REVIEW

4.1 Etiology and taxonomy

The *Aspergillus* genus is probably the most common group of fungi in the human environment, and people are often exposed to its spores (CABRAL et al., 2009). The species that make up this genus are filamentous fungi described as cosmopolitan, saprophytic, with a worldwide distribution and which can be found in very diverse environments, being able to colonise various substrates and can be isolated from soil, water, vegetation, decomposing material and air (FERNANDES, 2012; PRAKASH; JHA, 2014; SAMSON et al., 2014).

The genus *Aspergillus* is located in the Kingdom *Fungi,* phylum *Ascomycota,* order *Eurotiales* and family *Trichocomaceae.* This genus is made up of around 339 species, of which around 20 are considered potentially pathogenic, causing opportunistic infections in humans (SAMSON et al., 2014; PRAKASH; JHA, 2014). *Aspergillus fumigatus* is the aetiological agent that appears in first place as the most responsible for diagnosed invasive aspergillosis, and is followed by Aspergillus *flavus, Aspergillus niger, Aspergillus terreus* and less frequently by *Aspergillus nidulans* (BINDER; LASS-FLÒRL, 2013; PAULUSSEN et al., 2016).

Normally, the identification of filamentous fungi is carried out according to their morphology, so the identification of *Aspergillus is* based on the evaluation of their macromorphology and micromorphology, observing their characteristics such as: colony colouration, pigmentation of the culture medium, mycelial growth rate, colony texture and spore-producing structures (BALAJEE; MARR, 2006; BALAJEE et al., 2007).

As far as the macroscopic aspect is concerned, the main characteristic for differentiating *Aspergillus* spp. is the colour of the colonies, where they have a white surface in the initial stage of maturation, and depending on the species, their colour can evolve to various shades of green, yellow, brown, white, black or grey. The obverse side is usually white, golden or brownish. The texture of the colony appears cottony, becoming powdery or sandy with the production of spores, which may have rough walls, an equally important characteristic for species identification (KLICH, 2002; LACAZ et al., 2002; SIDRIM; ROCHA, 2004; MURRAY et al., 2010).

On microscopic observation, these fungi have septate, hyaline hyphae, with dichotomous branching forming 45° angles, where the asexual reproduction structures (conidia) are present, situated at the top of a terminal vesicle that arises from the extension of the conidiophore. The vesicle is covered by one or two layers of specialised cells and conidia, which are formed asexually and in interconnected chains. These cells that form the conidia are called conidiogenous cells or phialides, and their conidiogenesis is of the phialidic blastic type. When the thylakoid is inserted directly into the vesicle, it is called a uniseriate *Aspergillus* (figure 1). If there is a second layer of cells connecting the phialides to the vesicle, the *Aspergillus* is referred to as bisseriate and this is called metula (figure 1). (KLICH, 2002; MINAMI, 2003; MURRAY et al, 2010; GUARRO; XAVIER; SEVERO, 2010).

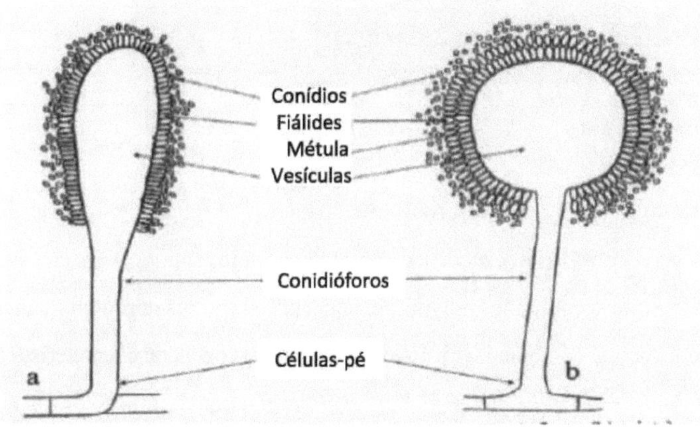

Figure 1 - Conidiophores of (a) *Aspergillus clavatus* (uniseriate) and (b) *Aspergillus flavus* (biseriate).

Source: adapted from Klich (2002).

Aspergillus species reproduce mostly asexually, so it is their asexual form of reproduction whose morphology is very characteristic that allows them to be identified microscopically, based on the morphology of asexual reproductive structures. Characteristics such as the size and shape of the conidial head, the vesicle, the arrangement of the conidia on the outside of the vesicle, the presence and shape of uniseriate or biseriate phialides, as well as the size and colour of the conidia are observed (BALAJEE; MARR, 2006; BALAJEE et al, 2007).

Even so, a few species are able to reproduce sexually. These teleomorphic states are characterised by having a closed, spherical structure called a cleistothecium, which contains the ascus containing the ascospores (figure 2). *Aspergillus* teleomorphs belong to the phylum *Ascomycota,* order *Eurotiales* and family *Trichomaceae* and are included in the genera *Chaetosartorya, Dichlaena, Emericella, Eurotium, Fennellia, Hemicarpenteles, Neosartorya, Petromyces, Sclerocleista and Warcupiella* (ABARCA, 2000; GUGNANI, 2003; PITT; SAMSON, 2007).

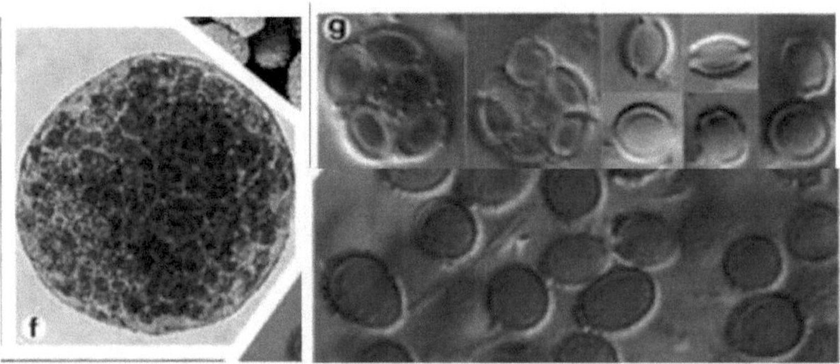

Figure 2-Microscopy of *Aspergillus glaucus*
F: Cleistothecium G: Asci and ascospores

Source: Taken from Hoog, (2000).

However, due to advances in molecular tools, the taxonomy of fungi belonging to the genus *Aspergillus* has been considerably modified. Thus, the determination of species has often been revised, taking into account the "polyphasic concept" of species definition, which is based on genomic sequencing, combined with phenotypic and phylogenetic characteristics. Thus, *Aspergillus fumigatus, Aspergillus flavus* and *Aspergillus niger* have come to be treated as complexes or sections, where several species are introduced, with different pathogenic potentials and antifungal drug susceptibility profiles. Thus, *Aspergillus* section *Fumigati, Aspergillus* section *Flavi* and *Aspergillus* section *Nigri* are nomenclatures that are being used in the literature (BULPA et al., 2007; GUARRO; XAVIER; SEVERO, 2010; GONÇALVES, 2011; JOHNSON; BORMAN, 2010; DEAK; BALAJEE, 2010).

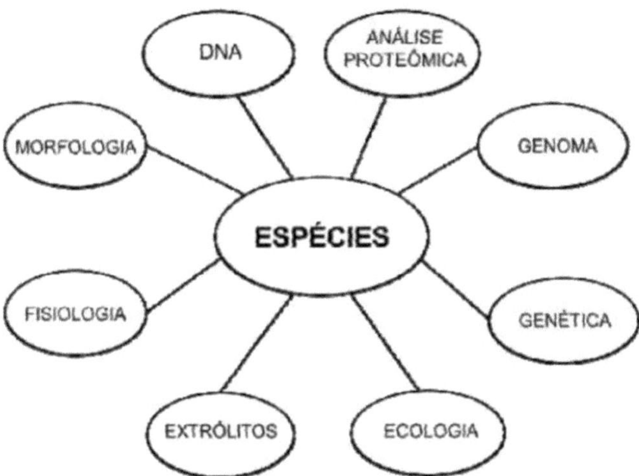

Figure 3-Scheme showing the integration of different characteristics that can be combined for a polyphasic taxonomic classification of an *Aspergillus* species

Source: Samson, Hong and Frisvad (2006) adapted and updated.

4.1.1 Aspergillus section *Fumigati*

Morphologically, the species of the *A. fumigatus* complex belong to the subgenus *Fumigati,* section *Fumigati*, and can be identified macroscopically by their fast-growing colonies (5-7 cm after 10 days at 28°C), where at the start of development, on Czapek agar (CZ) medium, they have a white colour, which over the days turns bluish green or greyish blue, with a cream, yellow, dark green or dark brown reverse. On microscopic analysis, they have columnar conidial heads with balloon-shaped vesicles and uniseriate phialides, smooth-walled conidiophores with globose to subglobose conidia, an olive green colour and a slightly equinulate surface (BALAJEE, MARR, 2006; PITT; SAMSON, 2007; SAMSON et al, 2007a, b, c).

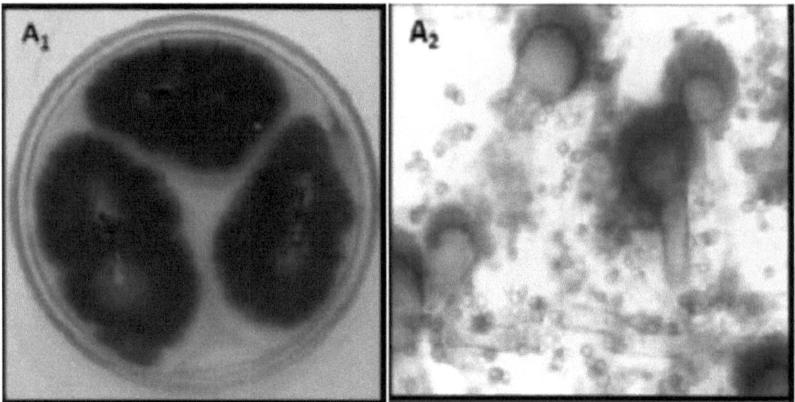

Figure 4- Culture of *Aspergillus fumigatus*
AI: 15-day-old cultures of *Aspergillus* fumigatus on Czapek agar at 28°C;

A2: conidiophores *of Aspergillus* fumigatus (lOOx)

Source: Brandão, (2012).

The members of the Fumigati complex show a coincidence of morphological characteristics between various species that are genetically distinct (BALAJEE et al., 2007), which makes it impossible to identify *Aspergillus* species by conventional procedures that are commonly used in clinical and environmental microbiology and without the polyphasic approach. Genetic and molecular tools involving the polymerase chain reaction (PCR), which amplifies the genes that encode 0-tubulin and calmodulin (NEDEL; PASQUALOTTO, 2014), analysis of deoxyribonucleic acid (DNA) sequences and phylogeny studies make it possible to solve the problems of atypical data arising from the large number of species present in this complex (ALCAZAR-FUOLI et al., 2008; SERRANO et al., 2011).

Some species that can be found in this section: *Aspergillus fumigatus sensu stricto and* its cryptic species *Aspergillus lentulus, Aspergillus udagawae, Aspergillus viridinutans, Aspergillus felis, Aspergillus fischeri, Aspergillus pseudofischeri, Aspergillus hiratsukae* (FRANCISCO, 2017).

4.1.2 Aspergillus section *Flavi*

The species of *A.flavus species* belong to the subgenus *Circumdati,* section *Flavi*, and in their macroscopic analysis, they show moderately fast-growing colonies (3.5-5 cm after 10 days at 28°C) or fast-growing colonies (6-7.5 cm after 10 days at 28°C), on CZ, which have a flocculent to granular appearance, casually show radial grooves, or a cerebriform appearance, yellowish green colour or, rarely, yellowish brown with a cream or pinkish reverse; also the production, in several strains, of dark brown to black sclerotia, especially in young colonies. Microscopic features include uniseriate and biseriate conidial heads, especially radial ones; spherical vesicles with metulae that occupy practically the entire surface; hyaline or pale brown stipes, with a rough surface, and globose or ellipsoid conidia, with a smooth or slightly rough surface (PITT; SAMSON, 2007; SAMSON et al., 2007a, b, c).

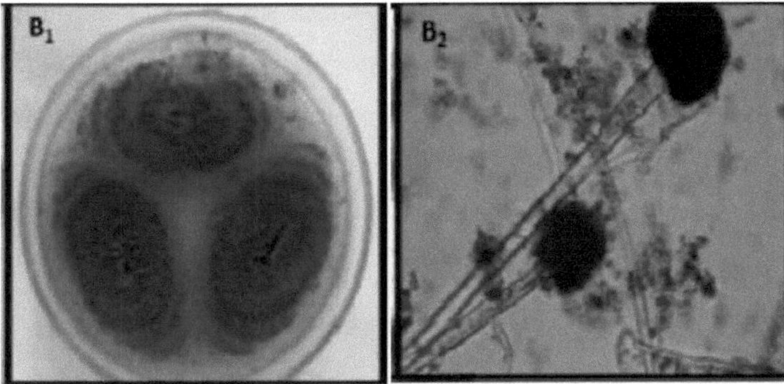

Figure 5- Culture of *Aspergillus flavus*
BI: 15-day-old cultures of *Aspergillusflavus* on Czapek agar at 28°C;
B2: conidiophores *of Aspergillus flavus* (400x)
Source: Brandão (2012).

A. flavus has a wide geographical distribution, as do other *Aspergillus* species, especially in cultivated areas. It is a saprophytic fungus capable of surviving on various sources of organic nutrients, such as trees, decaying wood, cotton, animal fodder, compost heaps, animal corpses and stored grain (HEDAYATI et al., 2007).

These fungi are producers of aflatoxins, natural carcinogens and cyclopiazonic acid, which is toxic to a large number of animals and humans (YU et al., 2005; HEDAYATI et al., 2007).

Next to *A. fumigatus, A. Flavus is* the second most common cause of invasive and non-invasive aspergillosis in humans and animals (DENNING et al., 2003). *A. novoparasiticus* (GONÇALVES et al., 2012), *A. mottae, A. Sergi, A. transmontanensis*

(SOARES et al., 2012), are examples of species belonging to this section.

4.1.3 Aspergillus section *Nigri*

Like *A. Flavus,* the species of *A. niger* belong to the subgenus *Circumdati,* but are classified in section *Nigri*, where they macroscopically present fast-growing colonies (4.5-6.5cm in 10 days at 28°C) on CZ, often with radial grooves, granular, initially white to yellow in colour, turning black with a cream or pale yellow reverse. On microscopy, they are distinguished by biseriate, radial conidial heads; spherical vesicles and metulae occupying their entire surface; thick-walled, smooth stipes, which can be hyaline or pigmented brown or pale yellow; and brown, globose or subglobose conidia with thick, ornamented walls (PITT; SAMSOM, 2007; SAMSOM et al., 2007a, b, c).

This section includes several species of great importance in food mycology, medical mycology and biotechnology (SAMSON et al., 2007). Many of the species in this section are widely used in industry, for example for the production of organic acids, such as citric and gluconic acids, which are produced *by Aspergillus* niger (ABARCA et al., 2004).

Some of the fungi belonging to this section are: A. eucalypticola, A. fijiensis, A. indologenus and A. neoniger (VARGA et al., 2011).

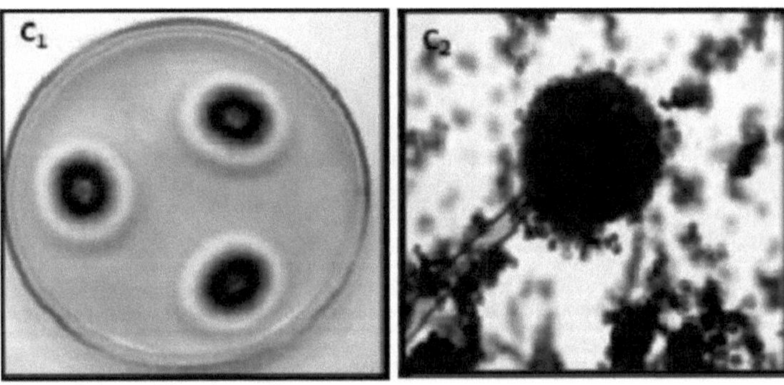

Figure *6-Aspergillus niger* culture
Cl: Cultures of *Aspergillus niger* (Cl) aged 15 days on Czapek agar at 28°C;

C2: Conidiophores *of Aspergillus niger* (400x).

Source: Brandão (2012).

1.2 Epidemiological aspects

The genus *Aspergillus* is distributed worldwide and in various habitats (SAMSON et al., 2014), with no geographical predilection (THOMPSON; PATTERSON, 2008). Most species can be found in water, soil, decaying plants, household dust, some foods, especially uncooked ones, and in some building materials, hospital environments, where improperly cleaned ventilation systems and water systems aggravate their spread (DIMOPOULOS et al., 2012; PARAMYTHIOTOU et al., 2014; SABINO et al., 2014; GREGG; KAUFFMAN, 2015; PAULUSSEN et al., 2016).

A. fumigatus is the aetiological agent responsible for approximately 90% of cases of aspergillosis; however, the number of other species causing the disease is growing, including *A. flavus, A. niger, A. terreus, A.* nidulans, and *A. ustus* (LAI et al., 2009; LASS-FLÔRL, 2009; ALANGADEN, 2011).

It is estimated that more than 200,000 cases of aspergillosis occur each year worldwide, with a mortality rate that varies between 30 and 95 per cent (BROWN et al., 2012). Studies have shown that 76% of patients present the lung as the sole focus of infection, characterising the invasive aspect of the fungus, and 10% of patients present evidence in more than one site of infection (STEINBACH et al., 2013).

In a study carried out at a university in Texas between 1989 and 2008, where autopsies were carried out on individuals with haematoncological problems, it was observed that there was an increase in the incidence of invasive infections caused *by Aspergillus* until 2003, but between 2003 and 2008, there was a decrease in the number of cases, due to the decrease in the autopsy rate, essentially due to economic problems, but the early diagnosis of invasive fungal infections in patients with malignant haematological disease, before death, may also explain these results. (LEWIS et al, 2013).

In patients with chronic obstructive pulmonary disease, the epidemiology of invasive aspergillosis (IA) is poorly documented, despite high mortality rates approaching 100 per cent (CORNILLET et al., 2006; ALANGADEN, 2011).

Studies carried out in the United States have shown a mortality rate of 80 per cent in bone marrow transplant recipients with aspergillosis (LIN et al,.2003).

In patients with acute leukaemia, the mortality rate is 30% to 40% of IA cases; in solid organ transplant patients, the mortality rate is 60% (MASCHMEYER, 2007; SEGAL, 2009).

In Brazil, data on the epidemiology of invasive aspergillosis in hospitalised patients is scarce, mainly due to the difficulty in diagnosing the disease at an early stage (XAVIER, 2008).

Many cases of aspergillosis are not detected before the patient dies. In addition, Brazil has a low frequency of pulmonary autopsies and, consequently, conclusions about the incidence of IA and the epidemiological condition are unreliable (XAVIER, 2008; SILVA et al., 2009).

4.3 Pathogenesis

Invasive aspergillosis is an opportunistic infection, where the disease and its progression are the result of both the growth and virulence of the fungus and the response of the host (DAGENAIS, KELLER, 2009).

Within this context, host-related factors play a major role in causing aspergillosis. *Aspergillus is* an opportunistic fungus that rarely causes disease in immunocompetent hosts, as the immune system eliminates the offending agent, preventing possible infection (PAULUSSEN et al., 2016). When the immune system is suppressed, the host becomes susceptible to developing the infection (RATHEE et al., 2013; WARRIS, 2014).

In the high-risk population, *A. fumigatus* has become the most frequent pathogen of invasive fungal disease, causing invasive pulmonary aspergillosis (IPA). It has become clear that the virulence of *A. fumigatus* is multifactorial, and that it has developed mechanisms to help it survive in the environment. These mechanisms include: thermotolerance, secretion of extracellular proteases and extensive secondary metabolism. Some of these factors also contribute to its survival in the human host, but contribute to the devastating results that are associated with API. (BEN-AMI; LEWIS; KONTOYIANNIS, 2010).

4.3.1 Virulence factors

Among the virulence factors associated with fungi of the genus *Aspergillus* is their high sporulation capacity, which can disperse from 1 to 100 spores/mm^3 in the air, which, together with their small size (2-3 pm), can easily reach the pulmonary alveoli by inhalation, making the respiratory tract one of the main routes of entry into the body and the lung its main site of infection (WALSH; REX, 2002).

Its conidia are well adapted for dispersal through the air due to their small size and hydrophobicity, allowing them to remain suspended in the atmospheric air for long periods. The ornamentation of these conidia, such as echinulate walls, observed in *A. fumigatus*, increases air resistance, improving dispersal; the pigmentation of these conidia also corroborates, making these structures remain viable for a prolonged period even in adverse conditions; (O'GORMAN, 2011).

The melanin found in *Aspergillus* species protects the conidia from adverse environmental factors, such as heat, ultraviolet (UV) radiation and pH variations, demonstrating a survival advantage in both the human organism and the environment, thus acting as an important virulence factor, as it compromises the immune response to the pathogen, thus constituting a fundamental factor for tissue invasion to occur (CHAT et al., 2010; LOUSSERT et al., 2010).

It has been shown that the loss of this conidial pigment in *A. fumigatus* and *A. niger* is related to a greater susceptibility to reactive oxygen species that are released by nuclear polymorph leucocytes and monocytes during the host's immune response (JAHN et al., 2000).

The germination of *Aspergillus* conidia at 37°C correlates with their pathogenicity, where *A. fumigatus* is more thermotolerant than other aspergillosis-causing species, growing well at 37°C and tolerating temperatures above 50°C. It has been speculated that this growth at high temperatures may lead to the expression of virulence genes that confer additional benefits, but evidence for this theory is lacking (ARAÚJO; RODRIGUES, 2004; DAGENAIS; KELLER, 2009).

In one study, a comparison was made between the growth of *A. fumigatus, A. flavus* and *A. niger*, which showed a correlation between germination rate and pathogen prevalence.

These species showed similar germination rates at temperatures up to 30°C, but there was a difference when the temperature was raised to 37°C and 41°C. At the latter temperature, *A. fumigatus* germination increased, while *A. flavus* germination decreased by 45%, while *A. niger* did not germinate. This shows that the ideal temperature for the growth of *A. flavus* and *A. niger* is around 30°C. The study suggests that temperature plays a crucial role in the selection of pathogenic *Aspergillus* species, with *A. fumigatus* being the species best able to adapt to extreme changes in environmental conditions (ARAÚJO; RODRIGUES, 2004).

The production of toxins, which are considered secondary metabolites, is another virulence mechanism of *Aspergillus.* The main mycotoxins produced by *A. fumigatus* are: gliotoxin, fumagilin, helvolic acid, fumitremorgin A and haemolysin Asp, the most relevant of which is gliotoxin (PAULUSSEN et al, 2016).

Gliotoxin modifies the immune response and is capable of inducing apoptosis of various types of cells. Its immunosuppressive activity affects neutrophil circulation and inhibits phagocytosis (SCHARF et al., 2012).

On the other hand, fumagillin and helvolic acid, as well as gliotoxin, in high concentrations, are ciliary inhibitors that act by decreasing their beating frequency (KHOUFACHE et al., 2007).

In addition to the substances secreted, extracellular enzymes are produced, which allow the fungus to damage some of the host's natural barriers in order to capture essential nutrients necessary for its perpetuation (GUARRO et al, 2010).

A wide variety of proteases are produced by *A. fumigatus*, including metalloproteases, alkaline proteases, aspartyl proteases, serine proteases and elastases, as well as lipase production (ALP; ARIKAN, 2008). These enzymes play a dual role, acting both in the digestion and assimilation of protein substrates, and as chemical tools paving the way for the hyphae to invade the host's tissues, thus acting as another virulence factor for the fungus (OKUMURA; OGAWA; NIKAI, 2004; DAGENAIS; KELLER, 2009; KRISHNAN et al., 2009).

4.3.2 Host risk factors

Prolonged neutropenia is usually defined as the most prevalent risk factor for IA and is often the result of highly cytotoxic therapies. Non-neutropenic patients, commonly those on corticosteroid therapy, such as allogeneic transplant patients receiving corticosteroids for prophylaxis or treatment of graft-versus-host disease (DAGENAIS; KELLER, 2009), patients presenting with haematological neoplasia, in particular with acute leukaemia, stem cell recipients, solid organ recipients, patients treated with high doses of corticosteroids, are also susceptible to IA (RICHARDSON; WARNOCK, 2003).

The infection can affect around 15.1% of patients who have received an allogeneic haematogenous stem cell transplant and 2% of those who have received autologous cells (BADIEE; ALBORZI, 2009). These infections affect 2-26% of patients undergoing bone marrow transplantation and between 1-15% of patients who have received an organ. (SINGH, 2005).

Other causes can also predispose to IA, such as diabetes, alcoholism, cytomegalovirus infections, parenteral administration of antibiotics (RAJA; SINGH, 2006) and AIDS (CUERVO- MALDONADO et al., 2010). Studies have reported cases of IA occurring after severe H1N1 infection (Wauters et al., 2012) and after the use of extracorporeal membrane oxygenation (PARCELL et al., 2014).

The onset of infection is facilitated by a number of factors, principally the number of inhaled spores and the decrease in immune defence mechanisms, where a decrease in the number or alteration in the function of alveolar macrophages and/or polymorphonuclear neutrophils is a determining cause in invasive forms (BELLOCCHIO et al., 2005).

Most patients with aspergillosis are male, although gender is not yet considered a predisposing factor; this can be explained by habits such as smoking and alcoholism, occupation and promiscuity (HSU et al., 2010; NAM et al., 2010).

Possible risk factors such as genetic predisposition and environmental factors have also been studied. Genetically, it has been observed, for example, that polymorphism in tumour necrosis factor-a (TNF-a) is associated with an increased risk of IA (CUNHA et al., 2013). High production of interleukin 10 (IL-10) has also been associated. In relation to environmental factors, it has been described that transplants that take place outside laminar flow rooms have an increased risk of *Aspergillus* infection and that the summer months are more favourable for IA to occur (KRIENGKAUYKIAT; ITO; DADWAL, 2011).

4.4 Clinical aspects

The term aspergillosis includes numerous manifestations that depend on the site affected, the severity of the infection and the immune status of the host. The upper airways, lungs and surrounding structures are the most frequently involved sites of infection, although *Aspergillus* infection involving various other organs has been reported. It is of the utmost importance to recognise the spectrum of invasive diseases attributed to aspergillosis, such as invasive pulmonary aspergillosis, tracheobronchial aspergillosis, chronic necrotizing pulmonary aspergillosis and invasive nasosinusal aspergillosis (THOMPSON; PATTERSON, 2008).

Invasive pulmonary aspergillosis (IPA) is the most common form of invasive disease. It is a form of pneumonia caused by *Aspergillus* spp, most commonly *A. fumigatus.* It is increasingly being seen in critically ill patients in intensive care units and in organ transplant recipients (WALSH et al., 2008; KOSMIDIS; DENNING, 2015).

Symptoms are very similar to those of other pneumonia-causing pathogens, often beginning with persistent fever, but this symptom is not always present in severely immunosuppressed patients, where its absence has been reported in cases of corticosteroid therapy. Other symptoms can include a cough, productive or not, dyspnoea and occasionally hypoxia. Later in the infection, haemoptysis and pleuritic chest pain can occur (GREGG; KAUFFMAN, 2015).

A careful history should be taken in those patients at risk of API, as they are usually unable to mount an immunological response and therefore do not show a febrile response. The symptoms of haemoptysis and pleuritic chest pain serve as a reminder of the angioinvasive nature of aspergillosis (THOMPSON; PATTERSON, 2008).

Tracheobronchial aspergillosis caused by *Aspergillus* spp. is considered an uncommon manifestation, in contrast to the involvement of the lung parenchyma (PATEL, 2010). It occurs in patients with severe immunodepression (KANG, 2011) and has a high mortality rate, reported in more than 70 per cent of cases (KRENKE; GRABCZAK 2011).

The terms invasive pseudomembranous tracheobronchial aspergillosis, necrotising tracheobronchial aspergillosis, ulcerative tracheobronchial aspergillosis, tracheobronchitis aspergillosis and obstructive bronchial aspergillosis have been used to refer to the same process, i.e. tracheobronchial aspergillosis (PATEL, 2010).

Its clinical presentation is variable and non-specific, which leads to its diagnosis being masked and delayed. The most frequent symptoms are cough, fever and dyspnoea, and haemoptysis is reported in 11.5% to 26.3% of cases (WU et al, 2010; FERNÁNDEZ-RUIZ et al, 2012).

Tracheobronchial aspergillosis can be classified into four different forms according to the bronchoscopic characteristics of the intraluminal lesions: type I - superficial infiltration; type II - complete layer involvement, a deeper form with cartilage involvement and airway destruction; type III - obstructive (with airway occlusion greater than or equal to 50 per cent by pseudomembranes, polypoid granulation tissue or necrotic tissue); type IV - mixed form (coexistence of two or more forms) (WU et al, 2010). Type II seems to be more related to greater aggressiveness and worse prognosis (WU et al, 2010).

Diagnosis requires bronchoscopic examination and is associated with unfavourable outcomes, as its recognition is often delayed (DUTKIEWICZ; HAGE, 2012). Characteristic bronchoscopy findings include: tracheobronchial ulceration, nodules, pseudomembranes, plaque or eschar. *Aspergillus* tracheobronchitis should be suspected in patients who present with suggestive imaging and haemoptysis or in patients with lobar atelectasis or unilateral wheezing, which results in thick mucus plugs containing *Aspergillus* that fill the central airways (PATTERSON; STREK, 2014).

Necrotising aspergillosis is an uncommon form of aspergillosis and its diagnosis is usually delayed due to its similarity to other lung infections, such as tuberculosis (CHABI et al, 2015).

It usually occurs in patients with underlying lung conditions, such as chronic obstructive pulmonary disease (COPD), sarcoidosis and mycobacterial infections. However, immunosuppressive conditions are also a triggering factor (SCHWEER et al, 2014; KOSMIDIS;

DENNING, 2015). It has a slow evolution, between one and up to three months, with marked pleitropic radiological characteristics (cavitation, nodules and progressive consolidation with abscess formation), showing visible hyphae in the destroyed lung tissue or inferred from microbiological investigations (i.e. positive *Aspergillus* antigen*)* (SMITH; DENNING, 2011).

Symptoms presented by patients include a prolonged and recurrent cough, dyspnoea, weight loss and, less frequently, haemoptysis and pulmonary haemorrhages (SCHWEER et al., 2014).

Invasive nasosinusal aspergillosis is a potentially fatal infection that frequently occurs in patients with immunodeficiency (BISWAS et al., 2013), in less than 4 weeks of the course of the disease (ARUNALOKE et al., 2009) and is often associated with API. Symptoms include fever, cough, epistaxis, nasal discharge and headache, and ulcerative lesions may be present. In patients with progressive disease, the infection can spread due to its proximity to the paranasal sinuses, palate, orbit or brain (DIAS, 2008).

Other signs suggestive of this disease are: asymmetrical facial swelling, proptosis and cranial nerve abnormalities (reflecting orbital disease or cavernous sinus involvement), palate ischaemia and bone erosion (SEGAL, 2009).

Infection of the maxillary sinus can lead to direct invasion of the palate, with necrosis and perforation of the oral cavity or perforation of the nasal septum. In the ethmoid and frontal sinuses, infection can extend directly into the veins that drain these structures into the cavernous sinuses, resulting in cranial nerve deficits and thrombosis of the internal carotid artery. Ethmoid sinus aspergillosis can also lead to periorbital infection and extension into the extraocular muscles and the eyeball, resulting in loss of vision (WALSH, et al., 2008).

Early diagnosis and treatment, which includes aggressive surgical debridement, antifungals and modifying risk factors, are essential for improving invasive nasosinusal aspergillosis (SÚSLÚ et al., 2009).

Although surgical debridement plays an important role in the management of invasive *Aspergillus* sinusitis and can be a form of cure, in some circumstances, extensive resections or repeated surgical debridements can increase morbidity and mortality among neutropenic patients. Advances in surgery for maxillary and ethmoid infection can be of great value and can avoid more disfiguring surgeries. Reversing immunosuppression is a key factor in the success of this infection and in preventing extension and dissemination to the central nervous system (CNS) (WALSH et al., 2008).

4.5 Diagnosis

Aspergillosis, especially in immunosuppressed patients, has never been an easy infection to diagnose, given that its clinical manifestations of infection are not specific, and even with the development of more modern methods it remains a dilemma (STEINBACH, 2013). Among the main factors responsible for this difficulty in diagnosis are: the lack of specific symptoms, the fact that there is rarely isolation of the fungus in individuals who are colonised and the lack of tests with the sensitivity and precision required for early diagnosis (LACKNER; LASS-FLÕRL, 2013). The lack of knowledge that new risk populations are emerging is also a factor that can delay diagnosis (PATTERSON; STREK, 2014). Alongside the difficulty in identifying symptoms is the occasional lack of them. The patient's history and risk factors must be taken into account (THOMPSON; PATTERSON, 2011).

The main criteria available for diagnosing aspergillosis are (DE PAUWetal. 2008):

- Biological criteria: direct microscopy, isolation, culture and identification;
- Histopathological evidence;
- Clinical and radiological evidence;
- Clinical characteristics of the host (such as neutropenia, fever persistent, among others);
- Immunological, serological and molecular tests.

Three levels of probability have been defined to aid the diagnosis of invasive fungal infections: proven, where a histopathological diagnosis is required, and it is not necessary to determine the presence of host factors or clinical factors; probable, where there must be the simultaneous presence of a host factor, a clinical characteristic and mycological evidence; and possible, when only host factors and associated clinical evidence are included, without mycological support (DE PAUW et al., 2008).

It is recommended that the diagnosis of invasive aspergillosis be made through concomitant cultural and histopathological examination of tissues or fluids. Only in cases where this is not possible should a molecular identification method be used (PATTERSON et al., 2016).

4.5.1 Laboratory diagnosis

The simplest method of diagnosis is microscopic observation of a sample, but this method is very unspecific and confusion with another filamentous fungus occurs very easily. Furthermore, there is no distinction between colonisation and infection (BARTON, 2013).

Histological examination is considered an excellent method for confirming the diagnosis of aspergillosis, but it is often not possible to obtain the sample.
feasible due to the invasive nature of the procedure and the patient's serious condition, which could jeopardise their health (BARTON, 2013; CADENA; THOMPSON; PATTERSON, 2016).

Diagnosis through culture is a simple and inexpensive method, however it is very time-consuming and less effective, as it depends on the quality of the sample and is also subject to contamination (SWOBODA-KOPEC et al., 2016). There is a significant possibility of false-negative results, especially in samples from patients who have already been given antifungal therapy or if the sample was not collected from the infected site. Therefore, a negative culture does not exclude the possibility of aspergillosis when this was the only test carried out. However, it is important to do this whenever possible, so that *Aspergillus* species can be identified and differentiated from other filamentous fungi (PATTERSON et al., 2016).

Immunological tests emerged in an attempt to respond to the need for diagnostic methods that did not require the collection of samples from the patient (CADENA et al., 2016). The Platelia *Aspergillus* EIA® ELISA test, which consists of a sandwich-type enzyme-linked immunosorbent assay for the detection of the *Aspergillus* galactomannan (GM) antigen, is used to make a non-invasive diagnosis of the infection. This test uses a mouse monoclonal antibody directed against the predominant epitope of the fungal cell wall antigen (STEINBACH, 2013). Although this method has the advantage of being non-invasive, it may not be the best option for late diagnosis, especially if antifungal therapy is already underway, as this will influence the sensitivity of the test (SWOBODA-KOPEC et al, 2016).

GM is a polysaccharide present in the fungal wall that is released into the host's bloodstream during infection (MIGOTT et al, 2017), and its detection has been shown to be a useful test for the early diagnosis of invasive aspergillosis, with a sensitivity of 94% and specificity of 98%, although it has shown a high level of false-positive results (~10-15%) (BADIEE et al, 2009).

The detection of (1->3) - 0-D-glucan is also a non-invasive and very useful method, even in patients on antifungal therapy (SWOBODA-KOPEC et al., 2016). This glucan is a polysaccharide present in the fungal cell wall and can be detected to confirm the presence of a fungus in the sample, however it does not differentiate the genus and is therefore not specific for *Aspergillus* (MURRAY et al., 2010).

Molecular tests, based on the polymerase enzyme-catalysed chain reaction (PCR), have shown great sensitivity, however they are not widely used due to the requirement for specialised equipment and standardisation of protocols (STEINBACH, 2013). A major benefit of using PCR is that, although GM cannot identify infecting *Aspergillus* species, PCR could be adapted for species-level identification and also possibly infer general antifungal susceptibility patterns (STEINBACH, 2013). Studies continue to be carried out on these methods and there is already some data demonstrating their benefit when combined with GM detection (CADENA et al., 2016).

Although PCR testing shows promising results, this method is not yet recommended for routine use in clinical practice because few assays have been standardised and validated, and the role of PCR testing in patient management has not been established (PATTERSON et al., 2016).

The Matrix-Assisted Laser Desorption/Ionisation - Time Of Flight Mass Spectrometry (MALDI-TOF MS) method is another fungal identification method that has been on the rise in recent years. The general principle of this method is the rapid photo-volatilisation and ionisation of a biological sample soaked in an organic acid (matrix) after bombardment by an ultraviolet (UV) laser, followed by the analysis of the mass/charge ratio (m/z) of the mass spectrum (MS) generated from the ionised sample after its journey through a flight tube. MALDI-TOF MS analyses the protein content of treated or intact cells of microorganisms in the form of a spectrum that is considered to be a specific fingerprint of a microorganism (COSTA, 2016).

4.5.2 Diagnostic imaging

Isolated radiological findings alone do not characterise the diagnosis of aspergillosis, but when associated with clinical and mycological findings, they are of great value. Radiography and high-resolution computed tomography (HRCT) are among the most widely used imaging techniques (DE PAUW et al., 2008; KOSMIDIS; DENNING, 2015).

Typical chest HRCT findings in patients suspected of having IA include multiple nodules and the halo sign, which is mainly seen in neutropenic patients at the beginning of the infection, usually in the first week, presenting as an opaque zone due to haemorrhage around the pulmonary nodule, which can evolve with cavitation, constituting the air crescent sign, another frequently found radiological sign (GOLDENBERG; PRICE, 2008; KOSMIDIS; DENNING, 2015).

4.6 Therapeutic aspects

The three main families of antifungals used to treat fungal infections are: polyenes, represented by amphotericin B (and its different formulations); azoles, with various derivatives such as itraconazole, fluconazole, voriconazole, posaconazole; and echinocandins, such as caspofungin, micafungin and anidulafungin (ALASTRUEY-IZQUIERDO, 2015).

The treatment of aspergillosis should vary according to the type of manifestation. Prolonged therapy should be carried out in cases of chronic necrotising pulmonary aspergillosis (PATTERSON et al., 2016). In invasive pulmonary aspergillosis, it is of great importance for a favourable prognosis that treatment is started as soon as possible (CADENA et al., 2016). In the treatment of invasive pulmonary aspergillosis, the first-line indication is voriconazole. Alternative therapies are carried out with liposomal amphotericin B

(PATTERSON et al., 2016). However, when aspergillosis affects the central nervous system (CNS), sometimes surgery also proves to be a good treatment (CADENA et al., 2016).

In patients who are using immunosuppressive therapy, it is extremely important to significantly reduce the dose of this medication, or even exclude it, when possible, before starting antifungal therapy. Treating aspergillosis concomitantly with chemotherapy, on the other hand, should be a decision assessed by various specialists, taking into account the conditions and risks of each patient (PATTERSON et al., 2016).

Amphotericin B (AMB) is an antifungal of the polyene class and has a broad spectrum of action that covers most filamentous and yeast-like fungi (KHAN; El-CHARABATYB; El-SAYEGH, 2015).

Its basic molecular structure is made up of a lactam ring, with a rigid lipophilic chain containing seven conjugated double bonds, and a hydrophilic portion (figure 7) (CARVALHO, 2013).

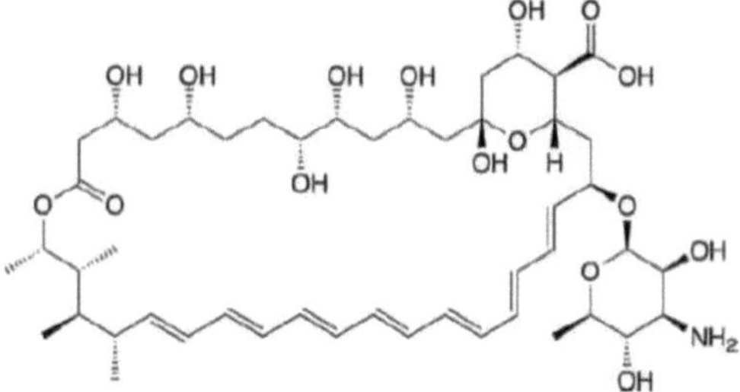

Figura 7 - Chemical structure of Amphotericin B

Source: Lewis (2010)

It is administered intravenously, as AMB is not absorbed orally (PATTERSON et al., 2016).

Its mechanism of action is fundamentally based on its binding affinity for ergosterol, the main sterol constituent of the fungal cell membrane which is essential for maintaining its integrity (LATGE, 2009). These bonds lead to the formation of ion channels in the cell membrane which destroy the osmotic integrity of the fungal cell membrane and lead to the loss of intracellular constituents and cell death (CHANDRASEKAR, 2010; MURRAY et al, 2010).

For the treatment of most fungal infections, lipid formulations such as liposomal amphotericin B are a better alternative to conventional amphotericin B, as they are safer and have equivalent or greater efficacy (HAMILL, 2013). The need to develop these lipid formulations arose from the toxicity of AMB, especially its marked nephrotoxicity and the reactions related to its perfusion (HAMILL, 2013; PATTERSON et al., 2016).

Voriconazole is considered the antifungal drug of choice for the treatment of invasive *aspergillosis*. It has a broad spectrum of action against most species of *Aspergillus* and many other filamentous fungi, and is used for opportunistic infections in immunocompromised patients (GREGG; KAUFFMAN, 2015; KHAN et al., 2015).

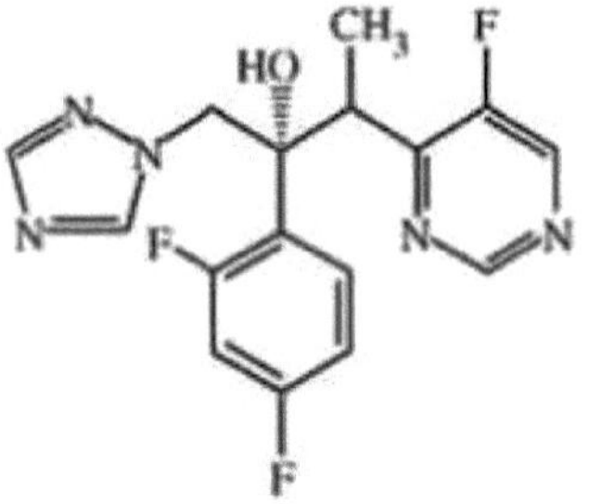

Figura 8 - Chemical structure of Voriconazole

Source: Thompson and Patterson (2010).

Its mechanism of action consists of interfering with the biosynthesis of ergosterol, which is present in the membrane of fungi, by inhibiting the CYP 450 enzyme 14-a-demethylase, which converts lanosterol into ergosterol. This inhibition results in an accumulation of toxic methylesterols and leads to altered growth and replication of the fungal cell membrane (THOMPSON; PATTERSON, 2010; KHAN et al., 2015; CADENA et al., 2016).

The recommended therapy begins with a dose of 6 mg/kg every 12 hours, twice only, followed by a decrease in the dose to 4 mg/kg every 12 hours. It can be administered orally or intravenously (IV). (KHAN et al., 2015; PATTERSON et al., 2016).

CHAPTER 5

FINAL CONSIDERATIONS

Invasive fungal infections have increased significantly as a result of the increase in the population that is more susceptible to these infections. *As* a ubiquitous fungus, *Aspergillus* is easily inhaled by humans, but rarely causes infection in immunocompetent patients.

The availability of new antifungal drugs in recent years has given clinicians more options, increasing the use of these compounds not only to treat the diagnosed infection, but also as prophylactic, empirical or preventive treatment.

Early therapy is fundamental for a successful outcome, however diagnosis remains difficult and knowledge of the clinical presentation and risk factors by healthcare professionals is highly necessary, as this knowledge can lead to greater suspicion on their part, thus enabling early diagnosis.

There is a need to continue researching and developing new methods, particularly for diagnosis and treatment, in order to overcome the difficulties that this infection still poses.

REFERENCES

ABARCA, M. Lourdes et al. Taxonomy and significance of black aspergilli. **Antonie van Leeuwenhoek,** v. 86, n. 1, p. 33-49, 2004.

ABARCA, Mª Lourdes. Taxonomy and identification of species implicated in nosocomial aspergillosis. **Rev Iberoam Micol,** v. 17, n. 3, p. S79-S84,2000.

ALANGADEN, George J. Nosocomial fungal infections: epidemiology, infection control, and prevention. **Infectious disease clinics of North America,** v. 25, n. l,p. 201-225, 2011.

ALASTRUEY-IZQUIERDO, Ana et al. Susceptibility test for fungi: clinical and laboratory correlations in medical mycology. **Revista do Instituto de Medicina Tropical de São Paulo,** v. 57, p. 57-64, 2015.

ALCAZAR-FUOLI, Laura et al. Aspergillus section Fumigati: antifungal susceptibility patterns and sequence-based identification. **Antimicrobial agents and chemotherapy,** v. 52, n. 4, p. 1244-1251, 2008.

ALDERSON, Joel W. et al. Disseminated aspergillosis following infliximab therapy in an immunosuppressed patient with Crohn's disease and chronic hepatitis C: a case study and review of the literature. **Medscape General Medicine,** v. 7, n. 3, p. 7, 2005.

ALP, Sehnaz; ARIKAN, Sevtap. Investigation of extracellular elastase, acid proteinase and phospholipase activities as putative virulence factors in clinicai isolates of Aspergillus species. **Journal of basic microbiology,** v. 48, n. 5, p. 331-337,2008.

APERIS, Georgios; ALIVANIS, Polichronis. Posaconazole: a new antifungal weapon. **Reviews on recent clinical trials,** v. 6, n. 3, p. 204-219,2011.

ARAÚJO, Ricardo; RODRIGUES, Acacio Gonçalves. Variability of germinative potential among pathogenic species of Aspergillus. **Journal of Clinical Microbiology,** v. 42, n. 9, p. 4335-4337,2004.

ARUNALOKE, Chakrabarti et al. Fungai Rhinosinusitis: A Categorisation and Definitional Schema Addressing Current Controversies. **QNRS Repository,** v. 2011, n. l,p. 3063,2011.

ASKEW, David S.; KONTOYIANNIS, Dimitrios P.; CLEMONS, Karl V. Advances against aspergillosis: biology, host response, diagnosis and treatment. **Mycopathologia,** v. 178, n. 5-6, p. 321-324, 2014.

BADDLEY, John W. et al. Aspergillosis in Intensive Care Unit (ICU) patients: epidemiology and economic outcomes. **BMC infectious diseases,** v. 13, n. 1, p. 29, 2013.
BADIEE, Parisa et al. Study on invasive fungal infections in immunocompromised patients to present a suitable early diagnostic procedure. **International Journal of Infectious Diseases,** v. 13, n. 1, p. 97-102, 2009.

BADIEE, Parisa; ALBORZI, Abdolvahab. Detection of Aspergillus species in bone marrow transplant patients. **The Journal of Infection in Developing Countries,** v. 4, n. 08, p. 511-516, 2010.

BALAJEE, S. A. et al. Aspergillus species Identification in the clinicai setting. **Studies in mycology,** v. 59, p. 39-46,2007.

BALAJEE, S. Arunmozhi; MARR, Kieren A. Phenotypic and genotypic identification of human pathogenic aspergilli. 2006.

BARBERAN, Jose; MENSA, Jose. Invasive pulmonary aspergillosis in patients with chronic obstructive pulmonary disease. **Revista iberoamericana de micologia,** v. 31, n. 4, p. 237-241, 2014.

BARTON, Richard C. Laboratory diagnosis of invasive aspergillosis: from diagnosis to prediction of outcome. **Scientifica,** v. 2013,2013.

BEISSWENGER, Christoph; HESS, Christian; BALS, Robert. Aspergillus fumigatus conidia induce interferon-P signalling in respiratory epithelial cells. **European Respiratory Journal,** v. 39, n. 2, p. 411-418, 2012.

BELLOCCHIO, S. et al. Immunity to Aspergillus fumigatus: the basis for immunotherapy and vaccination. **Medical mycology,** v. 43, n. supl, p. 181-188, 2005.

BEN-AMI, Ronen; LEWIS, Russell E.; KONTOYIANNIS, Dimitrios P. Enemy of the (immunosuppressed) State: an update on the pathogenesis of Aspergillus fumigatus infection. **British journal of haematology,** v. 150, n. 4, p. 406-417, 2010.

BINDER, Ulrike; LASS-FLORL, Comelia. New insights into invasive aspergillosis-from the pathogen to the disease. **Current pharmaceutical design,** v. 19, n. 20, p. 3679-3688, 2013.

BISWAS, S. S. et al. Acute invasive fungal rhinosinusitis: our experience in immunocompromised host. **Mymensingh Medical Journal: MMJ,** v. 22, n. 4, p. 814-819, 2013.

BRANDÃO, Ildnay de Souza Lima. Comparative analysis of laboratory methods for diagnosing pulmonary aspergillosis. 2012.

BROWN, Gordon D. et al. Hidden killers: human fungal infections. Science **translational medicine,** v. 4, n. 165, p. 165rvl3-165rvl3, 2012.

BULPA, Pierre; DIVE, A.; SIBILLE, Yves. Invasive pulmonary aspergillosis in patients with chronic obstructive pulmonary disease. **European Respiratory Journal,** v. 30, n. 4, p. 782-800, 2007.

CABRAL, Fernanda C. et al. Semi-invasive pulmonary aspergillosis in an immunosuppressed patient: a case report. **Cases journal,** v. 2, n. 1, p. 40, 2009. CADENA, Jose; THOMPSON, George R.; PATTERSON, Thomas F. Invasive aspergillosis: current strategies for diagnosis and management. **Infections Disease Clinics,** v. 30, n. 1, p. 125-142, 2016.

CARVALHO, LIC. **Aspergillus and aspergillosis - challenges in combating the disease.** 2013. Doctoral thesis. Master's Thesis, Fernando Pessoa University.

CHABI, M. L. et al. Pulmonary aspergillosis. **Diagnostic and interventional imaging,** v. 96, n. 5, p. 435-442, 2015.

CHAI, Louis YA et al. Aspergillus fumigatus conidial melanin modulates host cytokine response. **Immunobiology,** v. 215, n. 11, p. 915-920, 2010.

CHANDRASEKAR, Pranatharthi. Management of invasive fungal infections: a role for polyenes. **Journal of antimicrobial chemotherapy,** v. 66, n. 3, p. 457- 465, 2010.

CORNILLET, A. et al. Comparison of epidemiological, clinical, and biological features of invasive aspergillosis in neutropenic and nonneutropenic patients: a 6-year survey. **Clinicai Infections Diseases,** v. 43, n. 5, p. 577-584,2006.

COSTA, Ane Francyne et al. New approaches in the laboratory diagnosis of mycoses: the

MALDI-TOF MS system. 2016.

CUERVO-MALDONADO, Sonia Isabel et al. Update on Aspergilosis with emphasis on invasive Aspergilosis. **Infectio,** v. 14, p. 131-144,2010.

CUNHA, Cristina et al. Human genetic susceptibility to invasive aspergillosis. **PLoS pathogens,** v. 9, n. 8, p. el003434, 2013.

DAGENAIS, Taylor RT; KELLER, Nancy P. Pathogenesis of Aspergillus fiimigatus in invasive aspergillosis. Clinicai microbiology reviews, v. 22, n. 3, p. 447-465, 2009.

DE HOOG, Gerrit S. et al. Atlas of clinicai fungi. Centraalbureau voor Schimmelcultures (CBS), 2000.

DE PAUW, Ben et al. Revised definitions of invasive fungai disease from the European organisation for research and treatment of cancer/invasive fungai infections cooperative group and the national institute of allergy and infectious diseases mycoses study group (EORTC/MSG) consensus group. **Clinicai infectious diseases,** v. 46, n. 12, p. 1813-1821, 2008.

DEAK, Eszter; BALAJEE, S. Arunmozhi. Molecular methods for identification of Aspergillus species. In: **Aspergillosis: from diagnosis to prevention.** Springer, Dordrecht, 2010. p. 75-85.

Denning D. Introduction. In: **Aspergillosis: from diagnosis to prevention.** Springer, Dordrecht, 2010. p. 75-85.

DENNING, David W. et al. Chronic cavitary and fibrosing pulmonary and pleural aspergillosis: case series, proposed nomenclature change, and review. **Clinicai infectious diseases,** v. 37, n. Supplement_3, p. S265-S280, 2003.

DIAS, Viviane Maria de Carvalho Hessel. Invasive aspergillosis in haematopoietic stem cell transplant recipients. 2008.

DIMOPOULOS, George et al. Invasive aspergillosis in the intensive care unit. **Annals of the New York Academy of Sciences,** v. 1272, n. 1, p. 31-39, 2012.

DIMOPOULOS, George et al. Post-operative Aspergillus mediastinitis in a man who was immunocompetent: a case report. **Journal of medical case reports,** v. 4, n. l,p. 312,2010.

DUTKIEWICZ, Radek; HAGE, Chadi A. Aspergillus infections in the critically ill. **Proceedings of the American Thoracic Society,** v. 7, n. 3, p. 204-209, 2010.
FERNANDES, Natália Henrique. Production of xylanase and xylosidase by Aspergillus versicolor. 2012.

FERNANDEZ-RUIZ, Mario et al. Aspergillus tracheobronchitis: report of 8 cases and review of the literature. **Medicine,** v. 91, n. 5, p. 261-273, 2012.

FRANCISCO, Mariana Rato da Conceição Monteiro. **Characterisation of Aspergillus isolates from hospital environments: molecular identification and determination of antifungal susceptibility patterns.** 2017. PhD Thesis.

GOLDENBERG, Simon; PRICE, Nicholas. Opportunistic fungal lung infections. **Medicine,** v. 36, n. 6, p. 295-299, 2008.

GONÇALVES, Sarah S. et al. Aspergillus novoparasiticus: a new clinicai species of the section Flavi. **Sabouraudia,** v. 50, n. 2, p. 152-160, 2012.

GONÇALVES, Sarah Santos. Genotypic and phenotypic characterisation of clinical and environmental isolates of aspergillus section flavi. 2011.

GREGG, Kevin S.; KAUFFMAN, Carol A. Invasive aspergillosis: epidemiology, clinical aspects, and treatment. In: **Seminars in respiratory and critical care medicine.** Thieme Medical Publishers, 2015. p. 662-672.

GUARRO, Josep; XAVIER, Melissa Orzechowski; SEVERO, Luiz Carlos. Differences and similarities amongst pathogenic Aspergillus species.
In: **Aspergillosis: from diagnosis to prevention.** Springer Netherlands, 2010. p. 7-32.

GUAZZELLI, Luciana Silva et al. Aspergillus fumigatus fungus bali in the pleural cavity. **Brazilian Journal of Pulmonology,** v. 38, n. 1, p. 125-132, 2012.

GUGNANI, Harish C. Ecology and taxonomy of pathogenic aspergilli. **Front Biosci,** v. 8, n. 1-3, p. 346, 2003.

HAMILL, Richard J. Amphotericin B formulations: a comparative review of efficacy and toxicity. Drugs, v. 73, n. 9, p. 919-934, 2013.

HEDAYATI, M. T. et al. Aspergillus flavus: human pathogen, allergen and mycotoxin producer. **Microbiology,** v. 153, n. 6, p. 1677-1692, 2007.

HSU, Li-Yang et al. Galactomannan testing of bronchoalveolar lavage fluid is useful for diagnosis of invasive pulmonary aspergillosis in haematology patients. **BMC infectious diseases,** v. 10, n. 1, p. 44,2010.

JACOBS, Frédérique et al. An observational efficacy and safety analysis of the treatment of acute invasive aspergillosis using voriconazole. **European Journal of clinical microbiology & infectious diseases,** v. 31, n. 6, p. 1173-1179, 2011.

JAHN, Bemhard et al. Interaction of human phagocytes with pigmentlessAspergillus conidia. **Infection and immunity,** v. 68, n. 6, p. 3736- 3739, 2000.

JOHNSON, Elizabeth M.; BORMAN, Andrew M. The importance of conventional methods: microscopy and culture. In: **Aspergillosis: from diagnosis to prevention.** Springer Netherlands, 2010. p. 54-73.

KANG, Eun-Young. Large airway diseases. **Journal of thoracic imaging,** v. 26, n. 4, p. 249-262, 2011.

KAUFFMAN, Carol A. et al. (Ed.). **Essentials of clinical mycology.** New York: Springer, 2011.

KHAN, Asif; EL-CHARABATY, Elie; EL-SAYEGH, Suzanne. Fungal infections in renal transplant patients. **Journal of clinical medicine research,** v. 7, n. 6, p. 371,2015.

KHOUFACHE, Khaled et al. Verruculogen associated with Aspergillus fumigatus hyphae and conidia modifies the electrophysiological properties of human nasal epithelial cells. **BMC microbiology,** v. 7, n. 1, p. 5, 2007.

KLICH, Maren A. Identification of common Aspergillus specie. **Centraalbureau voor schimmelcultures,** 2002.

KOSMIDIS, Chris; DENNING, David W. Republished: the clinical spectrum of pulmonary aspergillosis. **Postgraduate medical journal,** v. 91, n. 1077, p. 403- 410, 2015.

KOUSHA, M.; TADI, R.; SOUBANI, A. O. Pulmonary aspergillosis: a clinical review. **European Respiratory Review,** v. 20, n. 121, p. 156-174,2011.

KRENKE, Rafai; GRABCZAK, Elzbieta M. Tracheobronchial manifestations of Aspergillus infections. **The Scientific World Journal,** v. 11, p. 2310-2329, 2011.

KRIENGKAUYKIAT, Jane; ITO, James L; DADWAL, Sanjeet S. Epidemiology and treatment approaches in management of invasive fungal infections. **Clinicai epidemiology,** v. 3, p. 175, 2011.

KRISHNAN, Suganthini; MANAVATHU, Elias K.; CHANDRASEKAR, Pranatharthi H. Aspergillus flavus: an emerging non-fumigatus Aspergillus species of significance. **Mycoses,** v. 52, n. 3, p. 206-222, 2009.

LACAZ, C. da S. et al. Treatise on medical mycology. 2002.

LACKNER, Michaela; LASS-FLORL, Comelia. Up-date on diagnostic strategies of invasive aspergillosis. **Current pharmaceutical design,** v. 19, n. 20, p. 3595-3614,2013.

LAI, Chih-Cheng et al. Current challenges in the management of invasive fungal infections. **Journal of Infection and Chemotherapy,** v. 14, n. 2, p. 77-85, 2008.

LASS-FLÕRL, Comelia. The changing face of epidemiology of invasive fungai disease in

Europe. **Mycoses,** v. 52, n. 3, p. 197-205, 2009.

LATGÉ, Jean-Paul et al. (Ed.). **Aspergillus fumigatus and Aspergillosis.** Washington, DC: ASM Press, 2009.

LEWIS, Russell E. et al. Epidemiology and sites of involvement of invasive fungal infections in patients with haematological malignancies: a 20-year autopsy study. **Mycoses,** v. 56, n. 6, p. 638-645, 2013.

LEWIS, Russell E. Polyene antifungal agents. In: **Aspergillosis: From Diagnosis to Prevention.** Springer, Dordrecht, 2010. p. 281-305.

LIN, Swu-Jane; SCHRANZ, Jennifer; TEUTSCH, Steven M. Aspergillosis case-fatality rate: systematic review of the literature. **Clinicai Infectious Diseases,** v. 32, n. 3, p. 358-366, 2003.

LOUSSERT, Céline et al. In vivo biofilm composition of Aspergillus fumigatus. **Cellular microbiology,** v. 12, n. 3, p. 405-410,2010.

MARTINS-DINIZ, José Nelson et al. Monitoring of anemophilic fungi and yeasts in a hospital unit. **Revista de Saúde Pública,** v. 39, p. 398-405, 2005.

MASCHMEYER, Georg; HAAS, Antje; CORNELY, Oliver A. Invasive aspergillosis. **Drugs,** v. 67, n. 11, p. 1567-1601, 2007.

MEERSSEMAN, Wouter et al. Invasive aspergillosis in the intensive care unit. **Clinicai Infectious Diseases,** v. 45, n. 2, p. 205-216, 2007.

MIGOTT, Gustavo Bellani et al. Clinical and epidemiological profile of patients with suspected pulmonary aspergillosis in a hospital in the state of Rio Grande do Sul, Brazil. **Revista de Epidemiologia e Controle de Infecção,** v. 7, n. 1, p. 34-39, 2017.

MINAMI, Paulo S. Mycology: laboratory methods for diagnosing mycoses. 2003.

MURRAY, Patrick R.; ROSENTHAL, K. S.; PFALLER, Michael A. Medical Microbiology (6ª). **Elsevier,** 2010.

NAM, Hae-Seong et al. Clinicai characteristics and treatment outcomes of chronic necrotising puhnonary aspergillosis: a review of 43 cases. **International journal of infectious diseases,** v. 14, n. 6, p. e479-e482, 2010.

NEDEL, Wagner L.; PASQUALOTTO, Alessandro C. Treatment of infections by cryptic Aspergillus species. **Mycopathologia,** v. 178, n. 5-6, p. 441-445, 2014.

O'GORMAN, Céline M. Airbome Aspergillus fumigatus conidia: a risk factor for aspergillosis. **Fungai biology reviews,** v. 25, n. 3, p. 151-157, 2011.

OKUMURA, Yoshiyuki; OGAWA, Kenji; NIKAI, Toshiaki. Elastase and elastase inhibitor from Aspergillus fumigatus, Aspergillus flavus and Aspergillus niger. **Journal of medical microbiology,** v. 53, n. 5, p. 351-354, 2004.

OLIVEIRA, Jeferson Carvalhaes de. Topics in Medical Mycology. 4. ed. Rio de Janeiro: Controllab, 2014. p. 95-102

PARAMYTHIOTOU, Elisabeth et al. Invasive fungal infections in the ICU: how to approach, how to treat. **Molecules,** v. 19, n. 1, p. 1085-1119,2014.

PARCELL, Benjamin J. et al. Invasive pulmonary aspergillosis post extracorporeal membrane oxygenation support and literature review. **Medical mycology case reports,** v. 4, p. 12-15, 2014.

PARTRIDGE-HINCKLEY, Kimberly et al. Infection control measures to prevent invasive mould diseases in haematopoietic stem cell transplant recipients. **Mycopathologia,** v. 168, n. 6, p. 329-337, 2009.

PATEL, Neelam et al. Tracheobronchial manifestations of aspergillosis. **Journal of bronchology & interventional pulmonology,** v. 17, n. l,p. 45-53,2010.

PATTERSON, Karen C.; STREK, Mary E. Diagnosis and treatment of pulmonary aspergillosis syndromes. **Chest,** v. 146, n. 5, p. 1358-1368, 2014.

PATTERSON, Thomas F. et al. Practice guidelines for the diagnosis and management of aspergillosis: 2016 update by the Infectious Diseases Society of America. Clinicai Infectious Diseases, v. 63, n. 4, p. el-e60,2016.

PAULUSSEN, Caroline et al. Ecology of aspergillosis: insights into the pathogenic potency of Aspergillus fumigatus and some other Aspergillus species. Microbial biotechnology, v. 10, n. 2, p. 296-322, 2017.

PERSON, Anna K. et al. Aspergillus niger: an unusual cause of invasive pulmonary aspergillosis. Journal of Medical **Microbiology,** v. 59, n. 7, p. 834- 838, 2010.

PITT, J. L; SAMSON, R. A. Nomenclatural considerations in naming species of Aspergillus and its teleomorphs. **Studies in mycology,** v. 59, p. 67-70,2007.

PRAKASH, R.; JHA, S. N. Basics of the genus Aspergillus. **International Journal of Research in Botany,** v. 4, n. 2, p. 26-30, 2014.

RAJA, Nadeem Sajjad; SINGH, Nishi Nihar. Disseminated invasive aspergillosis in an apparently immunocompetent host. **JOURNAL OF MICROBIOLOGY IMMUNOLOGY AND INFECTION,** v. 39, n. 1, p. 73, 2006.

RATHEE, Permender et al. Immunosuppressants: A Review. **The Pharma Innovation,** v. 1, n. 12, 2013.

Richardson MD, Wamock DW. Fungai Infection Diagnosis and Management, 3 Ed. Victoria: Blackwell Publishing Asia Pty Ltd; 2003. p. 166-200.

ROBBINS, Nicole et al. Hsp90 govems dispersion and drug resistance of fungai biofilms. **PLoS pathogens,** v. 7, n. 9, p. el002257, 2011.

ROTHER, E. T. Systematic review x narrative review. Acta Paulista de Enfermagem, São Paulo, v. 20, n. 2, p. v-vi, jun. 2007.

SABINO, Raquel et al. Molecular screening of 246 Portuguese Aspergillus isolates among different clinical and environmental sources. **Medicai mycology,** v. 52, n. 5, p. 519-529, 2014.

SAMSON, Robert A. et al. Phylogeny, identification and nomenclature of the genus Aspergillus. **Studies in mycology,** v. 78, p. 141-173, 2014.

SAMSON, Robert A. et al. Polyphasic taxonomy of Aspergillus section Fumigati and its teleomorph Neosartorya. Studies in Mycology, v. 59, p. 147- 203, 2007(a).

SAMSON, Robert A. et al. Diagnostic tools to identify black aspergilli. **Studies in Mycology,** v. 59, p. 129-145, 2007(b).

SAMSON, R. A. et al. The species concept in Aspergillus: recommendations of an international panei. **Studies in Mycology,** v. 59, p. 71, 2007(c).

SAMSON, Robert A.; HONG, Seung-Beom; FRISVAD, Jens C. Old and new concepts of species differentiation in Aspergillus. Medical Mycology, v. 44, n. SupplementJ, p. S133-S148,2006.

SCHARF, Daniel H. et al. Biosynthesis and function of gliotoxin in Aspergillus fumigatus. **Applied microbiology and biotechnology,** v. 93, n. 2, p. 467-472, 2012.

SCHWEER, K. E. et al. Chronic pulmonary aspergillosis. **Mycoses,** v. 57, n. 5, p. 257-270, 2014.

SEGAL, Brahm H. Aspergillosis. **New England Journal of Medicine,** v. 360, n. 18, p. 1870-1884, 2009.

SERRANO, Rita et al. Rapid identification of Aspergillus fumigatus within the section Fumigati. **BMC microbiology,** v. 11, n. 1, p. 82, 2011.

SIDRIM, José Júlio Costa; ROCHA, Marcos Fábio Gadelha. **Medical mycology in the light of contemporary authors.** Guanabara Koogan, 2004.

SILVA, Eduardo Felipe Barbosa et al. Chronic necrotising pulmonary aspergillosis. **J Bras Pneumol,** v. 35, n. 1, p. 95-98, 2009.

SINGH, N. Invasive aspergillosis in organ transplant recipients: new issues in epidemiologic characteristics, diagnosis, and management. **Medical Mycology,** v. 43, n. supl, p. 267-270, 2005.

SMITH, N. L.; DENNING, D. W. Underlying conditions in chronic pulmonary aspergillosis including simple aspergilloma. **European Respiratory Journal,** v. 37, n. 4, p. 865-872, 2011.

SOARES, Célia et al. Three new species of Aspergillus section Flavi isolated from almonds and maize in Portugal. **Mycologia,** v. 104, n. 3, p. 682-697, 2012.

STEINBACH, William J. Are we there yet? Recent progress in the molecular diagnosis and novel antifungal targeting of Aspergillus fumigatus and invasive aspergillosis. **PLoS pathogens,** v. 9, n. 10, p. el003642, 2013.

SÚŚLÚ, Ahmet Emre et al. Acute invasive fungal rhinosinusitis: our experience with 19 patients. **European Archives of Oto-Rhino-Laryngology,** v. 266, n. 1, p. 77, 2009.

SWOBODA-KOPEC, E. et al. Diagnosis of invasive pulmonary Aspergillosis. In: **Respiratory Treatment and Prevention.** Springer, Cham, 2016. p. 27-33.

THOMPSON, George R.; PATTERSON, Thomas F. Pulmonary aspergillosis. In: **Seminars in Respiratory and Critical Care Medicine.** New York: Thieme Medical Publishers, cl994-, 2008. p. 103-110.

THOMPSON, George R.; PATTERSON, Thomas F. Azoles. In: Aspergillosis: from diagnosis to prevention. Springer Netherlands, 2010. p. 7-32.

THOMPSON, George R.; PATTERSON, Thomas F. Pulmonary aspergillosis: recent advances. In: **Seminars in respiratory and critical care medicine.** © Thieme Medical Publishers, 2011. p. 673-681.

VARGA, J. et al. New and revisited species in Aspergillus section Nigri. **Studies in Mycology,** v. 69, p. 1-17, 2011.

Walsh, T. J. & Rex, J. H. Infectious disease clinics of North America. New York, USA, 2002.

WALSH, Thomas J. et al. Treatment of aspergillosis: clinical practice guidelines of the Infectious Diseases Society of America. **Clinicai infectious diseases,** v. 46, n. 3, p. 327-360,2008.

WARRIS, Adilia. The biology of pulmonary Aspergillus infections. **Journal of Infection,** v. 69, p. S36-S41, 2014.

WAUTERS, Joost et al. Invasive pulmonary aspergillosis is a frequent complication of critically ill H1N1 patients: a retrospective study. **Intensive care medicine,** v. 38, n. 11, p. 1761-1768, 2012.

WINGARD, John R.; HSU, Jack. Clinical Manifestations of Invasive Pulmonary Aspergillosis. In: **Aspergillosis: From Diagnosis to Prevention.** Springer, Dordrecht, 2010. p. 381-389, 2010.

WU, N. et al. Isolated invasive Aspergillus tracheobronchitis: a clinical study of 19 cases. Clinicai Microbiology and Infection, v. 16, n. 6, p. 689-695, 2010.

Xavier, M.O. *Applications and limitations of the galactomannan antigen detection method for the diagnosis of aspergillosis.* 2008. 104f. PhD thesis - Federal University of Rio Grande do Sul, Rio Grande do Sul, 2008.

YU, Jiujiang et al. Aspergillus flavus genomics: gateway to human and animal health, food safety, and crop resistance to diseases. Revista iberoamericana de micología, Barcelona, v. 22, n. 4, p. 194-202, 2005.

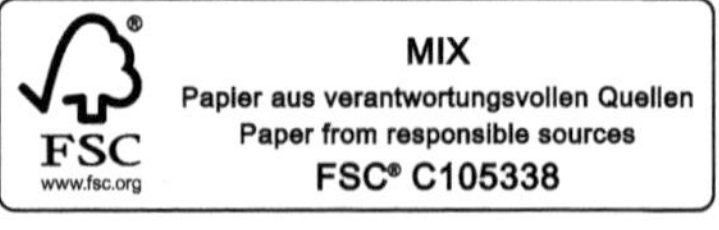

Printed by Books on Demand GmbH, Norderstedt / Germany